Mindful Yoga Therapy for Veterans Recovering From Trauma

VETERANS YOGA PROJECT

Suzanne Manafort and Daniel J. Libby, PhD

Published by Give Back Yoga Foundation, Boulder, CO

Published by the Give Back Yoga Foundation, Boulder, CO
for the Veterans Yoga Project.

The Veterans Yoga Project is a non-profit organization whose mission is
to provide education and support for the mindful use of therapeutic yoga
practices as an aid in the recovery process from post-traumatic stress and
other psychological difficulties among U.S. Veterans, their families, and
their communities. www.veteransyogaproject.org

Give Back Yoga Foundation believes in making yoga available to those
who might not otherwise have the opportunity to experience the transfor-
mational benefits of this powerful practice. We do this by supporting and
funding certified yoga teachers in all traditions to offer the teachings of
yoga to under-served and under-resourced socioeconomic segments
of the community and inspire grassroots social change and community
cooperation. www.givebackyoga.org

Edited by Patty Townsend, Rob Schware and Amy Lawson. Cover photo by
Lilla Szasz. Other photos by Eric Ramm. Graphic design by Susanne Murtha.

ISBN: 978-0-9888138-0-9

Library of Congress Control Number: 2012956568

Printed in the United States of America

23 22 21 20 19 18 17 16 15 14 13   1 2 3 4 5 6 7 8 9 10

Our Gratitude

We are so grateful to be supported by so many amazing, kind and generous people. We would like to acknowledge that support.

Thank you to Eric Ramm and Cathy Wong for your unconditional love and support.

Thank you to Patty Townsend for giving us a yoga home to learn and grow in and for teaching us your wealth of knowledge and experience. Thank you for all you have contributed to this project.

Thank you to Beryl Bender Birch for all your support, for being the mountain that you are and teaching us how it's done.

Thank you to Rob Schware for everything and more. You are the man!

Thank you to Robin Gilmarten and Bobbi Blake for encouraging us to go forward and giving us a healthy environment to work in.

Thank you to the Give Back Yoga Foundation.

Thank you to Sven, Kristina, Paul, Dan, and Gary for modeling the practices in the photographs.

Last but certainly not least, thank you to all Veterans and Active-duty Military Personnel for your dedication.

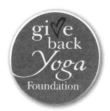

This project was supported and funded by the
Give Back Yoga Foundation

Table of Contents

Introduction

There is a look that crosses the faces of some veterans when they first hear about yoga for veterans with post-traumatic stress (PTS). The look says, "You've got to be kidding!" Often, another veteran will see that look and jump in, "I know what you're thinking and I felt the same way. It took me a while to even give it a chance, but you know, it really helps me with PTS."

Yoga is not a religion or a cult or a political movement. Yoga is a discipline and a practice. Yoga techniques have been in use for several thousands of years to train elite athletes, warriors, martial artists, and spiritual men and women. Many veterans, both those with and without PTS, are now using these techniques to build strength and resilience and to heal from the traumas of war. In fact, yoga is offered at many U.S. military installations and many of the PTS treatment programs within the VA nationwide also include some type of yoga or mindfulness practice along with traditional psychotherapy and medication.

What Is Yoga?

The term *yoga* has numerous definitions and may refer to a wide variety of traditions, practices, and disciplines. Yoga was developed several thousand years ago as a system of healing aimed at calming the fluctuations of the mind. Yoga in western....." and then at the end of that paragraph: "....and meditation. Practicing these elements is what leads to the calming of the mind. Yoga in Western healthcare environments usually refers to a collection of practices that has been adapted specifically based on the experience of veterans and active-duty military personnel coping with PTS and other mental and emotional distress. Yoga usually includes one or more of the following elements: breathing techniques, physical postures and mindful movements, guided rest (also called yoga nidra), and meditation.

What Is Mindful Yoga Therapy?

Mindful Yoga Therapy is a collection of simple but effective yoga practices that has been adapted specifically based on our experiences working with veterans recovering from PTS and other psycho-emotional stress. These practices can be used by anyone, regardless of physical or psychological limitations, to enhance the health of the body and the mind.

In Mindful Yoga Therapy, you will discover many different "tools" or "practices." You have many options in how you use them. While practicing meditation, for example, some people like to sit in a chair while others prefer to sit on a cushion on the floor. Some people prefer to practice breathing techniques while seated, and others prefer to lie on the floor. Mindful Yoga Therapy is about you finding what works for you. Many of the veterans with PTS who have practiced with us report better sleep, improved focus and concentration, less anger and irritability, and an overall greater ability to enjoy life in the present moment. Mindful Yoga Therapy has been especially helpful for veterans who are also participating in evidence-based psychotherapy for PTS.

This manual is based on our experiences with veterans coping with PTS and other trauma-related psychological distress. The practices in this manual, however, are effective for anyone dealing with stress. We present the practices in the form of a "tool box," in which you can find which practices are most helpful for you in various situations. We will go over each of these tools in this practice guide. First let's review what PTS is and how these specific yoga practices may help you better manage symptoms of PTS.

Post-Traumatic Stress and Its Symptoms

Post-traumatic stress, also called Post-Traumatic Stress Disorder (PTSD), is a debilitating condition that is triggered by a traumatic event. Traumatic events are dangerous and unpredictable experiences such as military combat, catastrophic accident, natural disaster, or sexual assault that result in overwhelming feelings of intense fear, helplessness, or horror. These events often involve risk of serious physical and psychological injury or death to self or others. Post-traumatic Stress reactions include negative changes in the mind, body, and behavior. Traumas such as these can shatter a sense of personal safety, disrupt life, and make it very difficult to trust others. Veterans with PTS may find that they avoid doing things or going places in which they are not in control of their surroundings. Sometimes there is also a fear of being overwhelmed by unwanted thoughts or feelings or being so afraid that the body will race out of control. Does any of this sound familiar to you?

There are three core *symptom clusters* of PTS. They are **hyperarousal**, **re-experiencing**, and **avoidance**. Let's look more closely at each of these.

Core Symptom #1: Hyperarousal

One way to think of *hyperarousal* is as a survival reaction. It keeps us alive! At the time of the trauma, hyperarousal reactions fortunately take over to promote our survival. These reactions, called "fight or flight," are activated automatically through the "emergency dispatcher" in the part of the brain that controls responses to dangerous situations. Instantly, your *sympathetic nervous system* brings a cascade of physiological changes that affect many parts of your body. First, breathing and heart rate spike. The pupils of the eyes dilate, or get bigger, to take in more light and visual information. Arteries, which carry blood away from the heart, also dilate, and veins, which return blood to the heart, constrict in order to increase efficiency of circulation. The body releases sugar, or glucose, the main muscle fuel for quick energy. Blood, oxygen, and glucose are rushed to the large muscle groups, enabling us to fight or run. Digestion and blood flow to extremities are slowed or halted. The body releases natural pain-killing hormones and constricts capillaries in case of injury. The emotions we experience during fight or flight vary, but typically include anger, fear, or a sense of exhilaration.

These and other physical and mental changes happen automatically and efficiently, again, to keep us alive. But here's the problem: having chronic PTS means that the sympathetic nervous system, or fight or flight, tends to be *overly* active even after the danger of the trauma has long passed. It is as if the emergency button has never been shut off. Many trauma survivors are *hypervigilant* and tend to overreact to people or situations that are *perceived* to be threatening even when they are not. Even many years after the trauma, there are people, places, or other things that trigger this emergency response even when there is no real emergency. Some veterans report that it is like "being constantly on guard" or that they are "always on edge."

The hyperarousal symptoms that result from an overly active sympathetic nervous system include having difficulty falling or staying asleep, feeling irritable or easily angered, having difficulty concentrating, being easily startled, and hypervigilance.

Hyperarousal Symptoms
- Feeling anxious, "on-edge", or on "high-alert"
- Difficulty sleeping
- Being easily startled
- Feeling irritable or easily angered
- Difficulty concentrating

Core Symptom #2: Re-experiencing

The *re-experiencing* symptoms include nightmares, flashbacks, un-welcome intrusive thoughts and feelings about the trauma, and in-tense psychological and physical reactions when reminded of the traumatic event. It is important to understand the connection be-tween hyperarousal and the re-experiencing symptoms of PTS. Daily stresses and sympathetic nervous system activation (fight or flight) can increase the frequency and intensity of these re-experiencing symptoms. Have you noticed that when you are really stressed out, on guard, or angry about something, you are more likely to have intrusive thoughts, strong feelings of distress, or flashbacks? This state may also carry over into sleep, with more frequent or severe nightmares in times of greatest stress. The re-experiencing, in turn, results in a "feedback loop" or what is sometimes called the *cycle of stress*. Hyperarousal leads to more re-experiencing, which leads to more hyperarousal, and the cycle continues.

Re-experiencing Symptoms
- Nightmares
- Intrusive thoughts about the trauma
- Physical reactions when reminded about the trauma
- Flashbacks

The Cycle of Stress

Re-experiencing

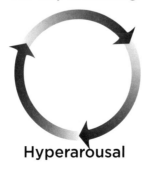

Hyperarousal

Core Symptom #3: Avoidance

Symptoms of *avoidance* include active efforts to avoid the thoughts, feelings, situations, memories or reminders of the traumatic event. This seems to a natural reaction; who wants to be caught up in this cycle of stress? Unfortunately, these efforts at avoidance actually make symptoms worse. Shutting down feelings at the time of the trauma made sense, right? There was not time to feel; it was all about reaction and survival! But avoidance and emotional numbing in your life today creates problems. While numbing may be familiar and comfortable, it also keeps veterans with PTS from living life more fully and connecting with friends and families. The use of substances is one way to numb feelings and to forget. Another way is to keep very busy or work long hours in order to avoid being still and having painful thoughts, images or feelings associated with the trauma. Some people may "dissociate" or check out mentally or feel disconnected from their bodies when under stress. Again, does any of this sound familiar to you?

Avoidance/Numbing Symptoms
- Efforts to avoid thoughts and feelings about the trauma
- Efforts to avoid people, place, and activities that remind you of the trauma
- Inability to have loving feelings
- Feeling detached or estranged from others
- Loss of interest or pleasure in activities
- Dissociation

How Can Yoga Help with Post Traumatic Stress?

In yoga class you will learn practices that will help you feel calm and in control. These practices work by decreasing sympathetic nervous system activity "fight or flight" and activating the *para-sympathetic nervous system*. The parasympathetic nervous system is sometimes referred to as "rest and digest" or "rest and repair," because the parasympathetic nervous system is the source of the *relaxation response* that allows the body to heal and repair itself. When the parasympathetic nervous system is active and the sympathetic nervous system is less active, the heart rate is slow and steady, the blood flow in the body is directed toward digestion and assimilation of nutrients, and the immune system is effective and efficient. The tools learned in Mindful Yoga Therapy will help you to learn how to activate the parasympathetic relaxation response during times of stress.

Mindful Yoga Therapy is designed in part to help you develop *mindfulness*. Mindfulness is a state of mind in which we experience greater clarity and focus. By developing mindfulness, or the ability to pay attention with interest and curiosity to this present moment, without judgment, we are able to respond more skillfully and in line with our goals and intentions.

Finally, Mindful Yoga Therapy is also designed to help you develop a sense of acceptance. Instead of avoiding uncomfortable thoughts, feelings, and sensations, these tools will help you accept and experience these thoughts, feelings, and sensations in a way that makes them less overwhelming and more controllable. Instead of falling into the cycle of stress, learning to radically accept uncomfortable thoughts, feelings, and sensations will help you develop psychological strength and resilience.

How Can I Use Yoga to Help with Hyperarousal Symptoms?

The primary way that yoga helps to control the hyperarousal symptoms of PTS is through observation and control of the breath. The breath has a direct link to the parasympathetic nervous system; when the breath is slow, deep, quiet, and regular, the parasympathetic nervous system is strong and you feel calm and focused. When the breath is fast and shallow, or noisy and irregular, the sympathetic nervous system dominates and you may feel anxiety, anger, frustration, or depression.

There are four breathing practices described in this guide and on the accompanying CD, "**Breathe In, Breathe Out**," that will be described in more detail later. When you feel agitated, you can practice one of these—right on the spot! By practicing a little every day, you may gradually learn to "stand down" more often. As you notice yourself feeling less agitated and more calm, you may also notice that you can think through problems more clearly, focus better, and feel more in control of your emotions, including anger. Breath is also a key part of the mindful movement practice. This movement connected with breath helps you maintain a balanced nervous system.

Another practice, called *yoga nidra*, can be done sitting or lying down, and involves being guided through a conscious resting and awareness practice to help with relaxation. Some veterans find that practicing yoga nidra regularly helps improve their sleep. You can choose to use the accompanying CD, "**Deep Relaxation: Yoga Nidra with Patty Townsend**", which you can listen to privately for approximatly 20 minutes, ideally before bedtime. (Be careful not to undo the positive effects of yoga nidra by watching the news, drinking caffeinated beverages, playing computer games, or doing something too stimulating afterward.)

How Can I use Yoga to Help with Re-experiencing symptoms?

Any practice, including yoga, that quiets fight or flight activity and enables you to feel calmer tends to reduce re-experiencing symptoms. In other words, it helps break the cycle of stress.

All of the practices in Mindful Yoga Therapy can be used for *grounding*, which may help you deal with intrusive memories and flashbacks by returning to the present moment. Grounding allows you to learn to be mindfull. These tools will help you learn to be mindfully "present in the present—here and now." If you are in the present moment, you cannot simultaneously be distressed over memories or flashbacks or concerned about what will happen in the future. The ability to ground in the present moment becomes easier and more effective the more you practice it. During the breathing, movement, and meditation practices especially, you can continuously return your attention, with a sense of interest and curiosity, to the sensations of the breath occuring in the present moment. A surprising benefit of this concentration is that it gives us moments of peace and quiet. And if we are able to enjoy a moment, then we can learn to enjoy several moments, and several more. Practicing all the yoga tools in this guide will help you break the cycle of stress.

How Can I Use Yoga to Help with Avoidance Symptoms?

Yoga may help you to observe and safely experience your own thoughts and feelings and learn to notice them without becoming distressed or overwhelmed. Instead of avoiding thoughts, feelings, and sensations, you will be invited to accept them as they arise with an attitude of non-judgment. Instead of avoiding people, places, and situations that previously created hyperarousal, you will learn to tolerate and accept what arises with an attitude of strength and confidence. By taking the risk to try yoga practices, you are already taking a conscious step to deal with your symptoms of avoidance.

It may be something new for you to notice whatever thoughts and feelings may come up and not run from them, and to know that you can calm yourself down in that moment.

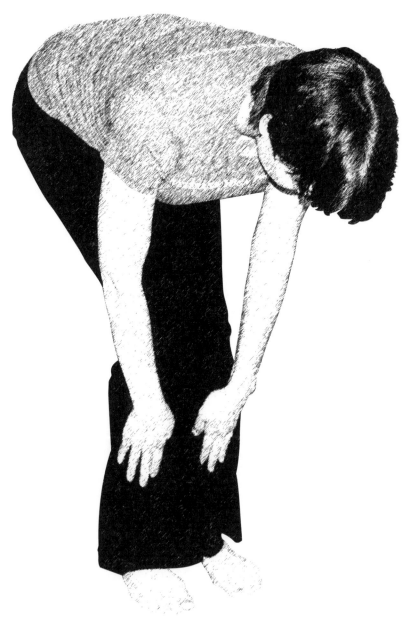

The Tool Box

The practice of yoga is thousands of years old and consists of a variety of different practices. The practice that we see most often called yoga in our society is usually just the postures and movement practices or *asana*. The ancient practice of yoga can include much more that that. There are also breathing practices, yoga nidra (a resting practice), meditation, and others.

Because we are all individuals, some practices work better for some people and some of the symptoms of PTS than others. With this in mind, we present these practices as a *Tool Box* with a set of individual tools in it that are always available to you. We invite you to try each of these tools and practice those you find helpful. You may want to try different tools at different times.

Yoga is taught by many teachers in the language of Sanskrit. We have added the original Sanskrit names for some of these practices in parentheses below. We present the original Sanskrit names of each of the practices in parentheses below.

The Tool Box consists of:

Breathing (Pranayama)
    Cellular Breath
    Three-part Breath
    Victorious Breath (Ujjayi)
    Alternate-nostril Breath (Nadhi Shodhana)

Mindful movement connected with breath (Asana)

Yoga Nidra

Meditation

Gratitude

This practice guide will address and explain each of these practices separately.

Breathing Practices (Pranayama)

The breath is where it begins. Connection with the breath is the backbone of any yoga practice and may be the most important gift you can give yourself.

We intuitively know that breath is the key to helping us find our way to comfort, calmness, and wellbeing. When someone becomes anxious or is in a stressful situation, we say "take a breath" or "breathe."

Our hearts beat continuously, our gastro-intestinal tracts digest our food, our kidneys filter our blood and control our blood pressure, our hair and nails grow, our skin protects, our immune system fights infections and disease, our liver helps clean our blood as it moves through our body, and all of these organs and systems work together to keep us alive and well. And we have little or no conscious control over any of it! Respiration is really the only basic physiological function that is under both conscious and unconscious control. If we don't think about breathing, we breathe. If we think about breathing, we breathe.

We can do things to make these parts work better, such as exercising and eating right, but we can't just stop our heartbeat. We can't increase the rate at which we digest food with just conscious thought. **_We can, however, control our breath._** Our ability to control our breath, or the rate at which we breathe and how deeply we breathe, is intricately tied to our ability to exert control over our thoughts, feelings, and behaviors. Essentially, we can use our breathing practices to help regulate how we feel and move through the world. Our ability to use breath in this way is a uniquely human quality.

Again, breathing techniques are used to cleanse, calm, and strengthen the nervous system, and thus increase vitality. Breathing is commonly used as an anxiety management technique. Breathing practices are also used as a tool to cultivate greater mental

14

control over our emotions and our reactions to them. The use of slow and conscious breathing balances the nervous system, initiates the relaxation response and grounds us. The nervous system is further balanced as we use our breath in coordination with the yoga postures and movements. Breath can be a bridge between the body and mind.

Although these practices are subtle, they are very powerful. We recommend that all the practices be done as nose breathing only, with your mouth closed.

We will explore:

Cellular Breath
Cellular Breath is a wonderful journey inward that allows us to stay present and grounded. It also allows us to find the healing qualities of the breath. We become able to feel how our whole body is actually breathing as every cell receives oxygen from the breath.

Three-part Breath
Three-part Breath helps us bring more breath into our body, allowing us to calm our nervous system and find a more peaceful and perhaps a more restful place. Breath is energy, and Three-part Breath helps to ensure that we are getting all the fresh life force and vitality we need into our bodies with the breath. It is not unusual to find that some people in our society are only using the top portion of their lungs. This practice teaches us to use the entire lung, which allows more breath to move through the whole body.

Alternate-nostril Breath (Nadhi Shodhana)
Science shows us that initiating breath in nostrils individually can help to balance the parasympathetic and sympathetic nervous system. *Alternate-nostril Breath* can be a profoundly soothing practice.

Victorious Breath (Ujjayi)

It has been said that this *Victorious Breath* strengthens and tones the nervous system. This practice will allow you to sip the breath in and out more slowly and wash it through your whole body. This is the breathing technique we will use in our yoga postures practice. It is both enlivening and soothing. The overall effect is deeply calming and centering.

Both the following pages and the CD that accompanies this guide, called "**Breathe In, Breathe Out**," will help you explore and learn these practices.

Cellular Breath

You may begin lying down with some support under your knees, such as a pillow or a rolled-up blanket.

Close your eyes if that feels possible. If not, just lower and soften your gaze.

Start by just observing your breath as if it is an exploration.

Notice how your breath feels today. It may feel deep and rich or it may feel shallow and light.

There is no right or wrong, so just observe. The purpose is to observe what today feels like, without judgment.

Bring your awareness to the base of your nostrils, right where the breath enters. Notice the sensation of it entering and exiting. Notice that it may be cool as it enters and warm as it exits. Allow yourself to feel this.

Draw your awareness in a little deeper and notice how the breath feels on the inside of your nostrils. Perhaps it is soft and fluffy, like velvet or cotton candy. You may also notice that your breath swirls its way in, and this may feel good. Take a moment here.

Now can you draw your awareness inward even deeper? Feel how your breath makes its way in through the nostrils and all the way into your lungs. Stay with this for several breaths. Maybe you can even imagine that the breath flows like a fluid as it makes its way in and then back out of your body.

Do you notice how your lungs expand when you inhale and condense when you exhale?

The next time you inhale and your lungs expand, imagine that the oxygen washes from your lungs into your bloodstream. From your bloodstream, the oxygen makes its way to all your organs and all your tissues and to every single cell in your body. Imagine that every cell in your body is expanding and condensing individually with each breath.

Just stay with these sensations and images and allow the breath to wash through you and nourish your cells, tissues, and organs.

If you like, you can focus on one specific area that may be troublesome. As you bring your focus to this area, treat your awareness as if it were a sponge. Every time you inhale, the sponge brings in new and fresh oxygen that washes through you and when you exhale it sends out the unneeded, unwanted or waste. This sponging can be used in one specific area of your body, or as full body awareness.

Take as much time here as needed.

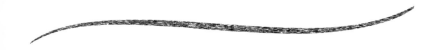

Three-part Breath

It may be helpful to know that our lungs are big, football-sized organs inside our ribcage. They have three lobes on one side and two lobes on the other. When we breathe we bring breath in from the tops of the lungs to the bottoms. For this exploration we divide the lungs into three parts on both sides and call them top lungs, middle lungs and bottom lungs. We will also explore bringing the breath to the bottom lungs first, drawing our attention upward to the middle lungs, and finally to the top lungs.

Please begin in a reclined posture, preferably on the floor. If you need some support you can place a bolster or rolled up blanket under your knees.

This exploration begins with just noticing your breath. Allow your-self to notice the inhale and the exhale. It is important not to judge the way you are breathing. You will learn to bring breath through your whole body as your practice continues.

Bring your fingers to the top of your collarbones and place your fingertips in the hollows at the tops of the collarbones. This is the top of the lungs. As you take a very large inhale see if you can feel the top of the lungs puff up under your fingers like a balloon inflating.

Next bring your hands to the middle of your ribcage or even under your armpits. As you inhale, see if you can notice how your ribcage expands three dimensionally as your lungs fill, and notice how they condense on the exhale. This is the action of the middle lung.

Finally bring your hands to your lower ribcage. As you inhale this time, see if you feel the expand and condense of your bottom lungs.

Now rest your hands down by your sides. Start Three-part Breath by just taking a natural breath (an inhale and an exhale).

The next inhale should be very slow. As you inhale draw your breath first into the bottom lungs, slowly bring it up to the middle lungs, and finally fill up as you bring breath to the top lungs. Then exhale fully. Take a natural breath.

Repeat four more times, being mindful to take a natural breath between each Three-part Breath.

After completing five Three-part Breaths, close your eyes for a moment and notice how you feel. Compare this to how you felt before you started the practice.

Alternate-nostril Breathing (Nadi Shodhana)

Science has shown us that we breathe dominantly in one nostril over the other and that the dominant side changes throughout the day. Alternate-nostril Breathing practice, or Nadi Shodhana, helps us breathe through both nostrils at the same time. Finding balance in the breath lets us find balance in the parasympathetic and sympathetic nervous system.

This practice may be done reclined or seated. Find a comfortable place. If you are seated, plant your feet firmly on the earth. Close your eyes if that feels comfortable, but if it doesn't just try to lower your eyes and soften your gaze.

This practice begins again with just noticing the breath. This is always a great place to start. You may notice that it is repeated at the beginning of each practice. It's a great checking in point. How does my breath feel today? It allows you to settle in and there is a bit of comfort in your breath's own unique rhythm.

Take a few natural inhales and exhales with your mouth closed. Then take a large inhale and exhale fully though both nostrils. Feel the sensation of the breath in your nostrils.

Now, take your awareness primarily to your right nostril. The next inhale will be initiated in your right nostril. Allow your awareness to cross over the bridge of your nose and exhale through the left nostril.

Your next inhale will be felt in your left nostril. Cross over the bridge of your nose and exhale through your right nostril.

This is one complete round. Remember, all you need to do is shift sides after each inhalation.

Try beginning your practice with five to ten rounds.

Allow yourself to come back to natural breath and notice the effects of this practice. You may notice that you are breathing through both nostrils at the same time.

Take a few minutes to feel the results of this practice.

Victorious Breath (Ujjayi)

Victorious Breath or Ujjayi practice can be done several ways. It can be used as a strong, powerful, and heating breath or it can be done in a soft, slow, steady, calming way. We will be doing a soft version.

You will also be trying to create evenness in your breath. For example you may notice that your inhale is a little shorter than your exhale. Or that your exhale is slightly more exaggerated than your inhale. In this practice you will be trying to even out the inhale and exhale.

This practice is done with your mouth closed and a bit of constriction is created in the back of the throat. It has an audible sound to it. It is sometimes referred to as ocean breath.

Start this exploration by imagining that you have a mirror in your hand. If you were going breathe on that mirror with the intention of fogging it up, you might open your mouth and breath on the mirror with a sound that sounds like ......HA.

Now, try this again, but this time close your mouth in the middle of the breath, and you may feel a bit of constriction at the back of your throat that creates a soft, audible sound.

Can you now do that with your mouth closed and do it on both your inhale and exhale?

Once this is established, start breathing with this soft sound and pay attention to the length of your inhale and exhale. Begin to create balance in the two.

Take a few moments to just breathe.

This breath can be taken with you wherever you go. It is a great tool to use in times of stress or anxiety. It will keep you present in this very moment and create a calming effect.

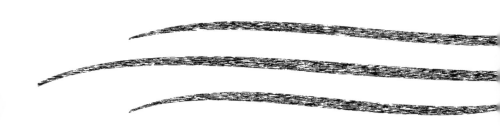

Mindful Movement and Postures (Asana)

Asana, or postures combined with mindful movement and breath, is the practice almost everyone thinks of when they think of "yoga." This ancient practice is full of wisdom. Although the side effects of asana will give you strong muscles and keep you in shape, there is so much more to this practice than just physical exercise.

In the tradition of Embodyoga, which is the foundation of Mindful Yoga Therapy, there are several principles that seem to aid in the recovery of PTS when accompanied by psychotherapy.

Support Precedes Action

We begin with *support precedes action* because support precedes any effective movement, non-movement or action. It is important to know that you have the support you need before you make any move forward, take your next step in life, or even just move into a yoga posture. In other words, support precedes everything! We have provided specific postures and techniques to help you find a connection to earth with your feet and even your hands when they are on the earth. The grounding connection to earth lets you know that you have the support that you need to move forward safely and with stability. This earthy, grounded feeling provides steadiness, a calm presence, and a sense of ease. With continued practice you may find new sensations of having support under you in many different areas of your body. You may begin to spontaneously initiate movement from these supports. When you know where your support is coming from, you find more comfort. This concept may apply in many areas of life—and we know it applies in our yoga practice.

Finding this connection, or relationship with earth, may help you begin to find a renewed relationship with yourself as well. Finding and nurturing this relationship with yourself, and feeling fully supported by the earth under you, will allow you to begin to explore your relationship with others too. Yoga offers us choice in our actions. Each of us takes our own time in coming into a deeper relationship with earth, with self, and with other. There is no timetable except for your own comfort. You're the boss in this!

We present the following supports in alphabetical order. Each one is equally important.

Acceptance

Your yoga practice will help you learn to practice *acceptance*. Acceptance of what is and where we actually are—in our mind and body—at each new moment and each new day is an important principle in yoga practice. But it isn't always easy!

You may step on your yoga mat today and have an amazing practice that feels so good that you can't wait to do it again tomorrow. When tomorrow arrives, you may have an entirely different experience. You may have physical limitations that don't allow you to do the full expression of the posture. You may be tired, or just not in a good mood. In practicing acceptance of how we actually are and feel each day, we just proceed on with our practice. Acceptance does not mean stopping or giving up! It means that you accept that your practice is different each day and you continue on. You keep practicing. You accept that you have some limitations, but you do not let them stop you.

While this acceptance starts on your yoga mat, it will enter other areas of your life. There is freedom in discerning what you can change and what you can't and moving forward with that knowledge.

Breath

Breath is the primary support for everything we do. The use of slow and conscious breathing balances the nervous system, initiates the relaxation response and grounds us. The nervous system is further balanced as we use our breath in coordination with the yoga postures and movements.

We have given you four practices that can be used independently, but when you are practicing movement we ask that you use one in particular, the Ujjayi Breath. This breath should be done with your mouth closed. If you can't keep your mouth closed when you are practicing, this may be a signal that you are pushing too hard and need to back off a little. There should also be a focus on keeping the inhale the same length as the exhale.

Slow, steady, and even, with your mouth closed, is the way to breathe in your movement practice.

Calm and Supported Spine

Structurally, our spine contains and protects our central nervous system. With the practice of the *calm and supported spine* we facilitate healthy movement that doesn't disrupt the flow of the central nervous system or the health of the spine.

Imagine that you have a golden thread that runs right through the center of your body, from your pelvic floor to the crown of your head. Imagine that this thread is kept long and unbroken. You can bend forward and you can bend backward, but without loosening or breaking the thread. It stays long and strong. You can even spiral around it, but still it is unbroken.

Full Body Postures

You will explore the concept of *full body postures* in your asana practice. A full body posture means that you form a connection from your *feet to your head* and from your *hands to your tail*. From this connection of your feet fully on the earth, you follow the sensation of pressing your feet firmly into the earth and drawing your awareness upward, all the way through your body to the crown of your head. As you reach your arms upward, you follow the sensation from your hands all the way through you to your tail. Being mindful that the postures are full body postures and you are not just swinging your legs or arms around, you naturally begin to feel more connected to yourself and to your environment.

Each day that you step back onto your mat you find a little more of this support and integration and less fragmentation. This feeling of integration will bring you back to your mat day after day.

Navel Support

Imagine for just one moment that you or someone else has a supportive hand on your belly or right on your navel. Can you also imagine that this hand is very softly pressing inward to create support? Allow yourself to explore the sensation of how this would feel.

We will call this *navel support* and will ask that you try to maintain it throughout your practice. Navel support is very important because it maintains the integrity of your spine by keeping it long and ensuring that your lower back does not collapse. This support also teaches you to pay attention and helps to keep you in the present moment.

Yield—An Active Relationship with Ground

Yield or *grounding* is one of the very first supports we explore. Like everything in life, it's important to know that you have the support you need before you move forward. We have provided specific postures and techniques to help you find a connection to earth with your feet, and even with your hands when they are on the earth. This grounding connection to earth lets us know that we have the support we need to move forward safely and with stability. This earthy, grounded feeling, or yield, provides steadiness accompanied by a calm presence and sense of ease. With continued practice, you may find a new sensation of having support under you in many different areas of your body. You may even begin to spontaneously initiate movement from these supports. When you know where your support is coming from, you find comfort.

Finding this connection, or an active relationship with earth, may help you begin to find a renewed relationship with yourself. Finding and nurturing this relationship with yourself and feeling fully supported by the earth under you will also allow you to begin to explore your relationship with others. Yoga offers us choice in our actions. Each of us takes our own time in coming into a different relationship with self, earth, and others. There is no timetable except for your own comfort. You are the boss in this.

Yoga Props

It is not necessary to use yoga props to practice yoga. However, the use of props can be a very helpful way to enhance your yoga practice. In this practice guide we give you the option of using them.

Yoga Mat — Your mat is probably the most important of all props because it keeps you from slipping and sliding. Mats come in many sizes, colors, and textures. It all boils down to personal preference. You will be placing your feet, your hands, and sometimes your face on your mat, so it would be better to buy your own mat instead of using the community mats in the yoga centers.

Yoga Blocks —Your block can be used in many different ways. Support for your hands in standing postures, forward bends, and twists are a few examples. You may also sit on your block and use it for some inversion postures.

Yoga Strap —Your yoga strap can be used to help you reach your feet in postures when you are unable to. It can also help to maintain the integrity of a posture.

Blankets —Blankets can be used as support in many ways depending on the way that they are folded or rolled.

Cushions —Cushions are used to find comfort in a seated posture while practicing meditation or breathing practices. Some cushions are filled with cotton and some filled with buckwheat hulls.

A daily asana or movement practice is recommended; a few times a week could be a very good way to begin.

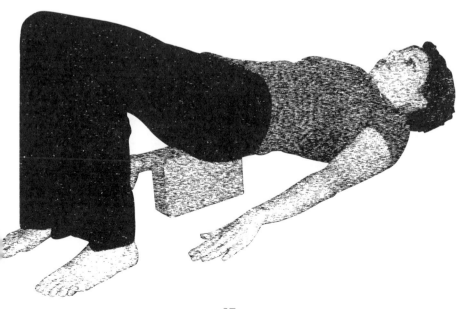

Mindful Movement or Asana Practice

Breathing

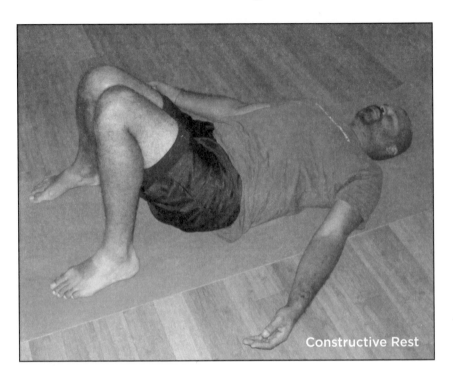

Constructive Rest

Begin by lying down on the floor in **Constructive Rest**. (Lay on your back with your knees bent and your feet on the floor hips distance apart. Allow your knees to rest together).

Continue here with one of the breathing practices (**Cellular Breath or Three-part Breath**). Spend about 5 to 15 minutes here. This is a good time to pay attention to being present and to notice that the breath is the tool to help you with that.

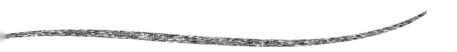

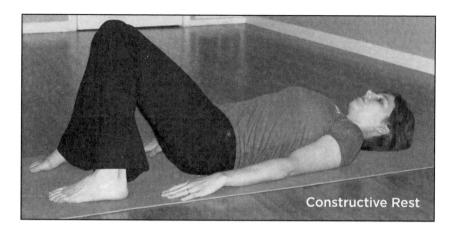
Constructive Rest

Moving Warm-up

Begin to use your **Ujjayi Breath** (see page 16).

Start your movement by bringing your knees hips width apart as you prepare for **Bridge**. Just notice your feet on the earth. Place your hands, palms down, on the earth by your sides. Press into the earth with your feet and hands. These connections help to ground you.

As you press your feet and hands into the earth, with an inhale lift your hips off the floor and come to the tops of your shoulders. Then with your exhale slowly lower down—one vertebra at a time—beginning with your upper back, through the mid back, and finally

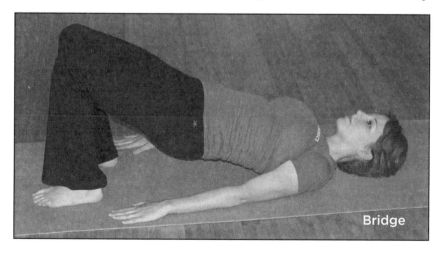
Bridge

your lower back and hips. *Repeat Bridge 3 times,* inhaling each time you press down to lift up, and exhaling each time you slowly roll back down.

On an exhale, bring your **Knees to your Chest** and give them a little squeeze. If it is comfortable for you, you may also roll your knees from side to side as you continue to inhale and exhale.

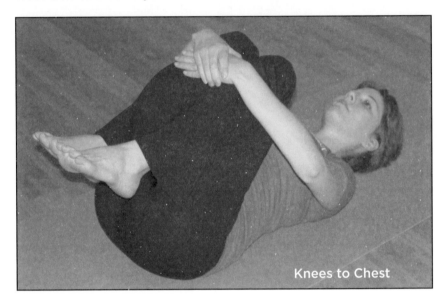
Knees to Chest

When you are ready, roll over to your side and come to your **Hands and Knees**. Place your hands slightly forward of your shoulders, and your knees directly under your hips. Bring your attention to your hands. Allow the hands to yield into the earth and let this keep you grounded and present. Softly bend your elbows and press the entire surface of each of your hands into the earth. As you press into your hands and connect with earth, see if you can feel the rebound of that connection all the way up through your body to your tailbone.

Next, imagine that you have your hand on your navel. Imagine that this hand supports you from the underside of your body. This navel support allows the spine to be long and supported, protecting and

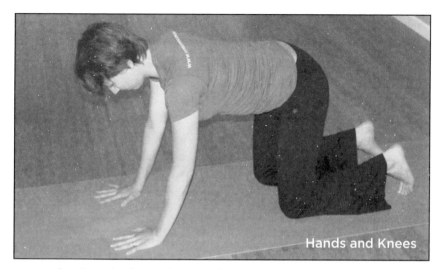

Hands and Knees

strengthening the lower back. We encourage you to maintain this support throughout your practice.

With an inhale, maintaining this navel support, **Raise Your Right Arm and Left Leg**. Reach them in opposite directions. Your hand will be reaching forward and your leg reaching behind you. Remember this is just an exploration. This is not about doing something right or wrong. Continue to explore your supports. The grounding

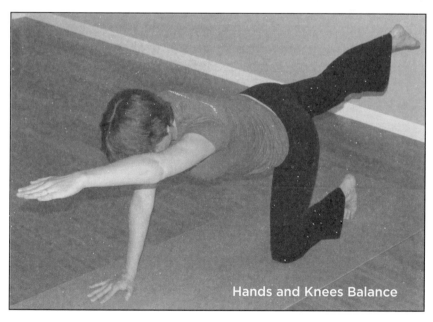

Hands and Knees Balance

of the opposite hand and leg that are pressing into the earth and the navel support should keep you steady and even. Remain here for 5 breaths and then exhale as you draw them back down and place them on the earth. *Repeat other side.*

Press your hands into the earth as you exhale and press back into **Wisdom Pose**. See if you can notice the even connection from the press of the hands all the way through to your tailbone. *Take 3 breaths here.*

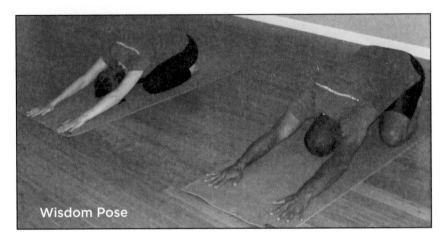
Wisdom Pose

Keeping your lower legs on the earth, inhale and draw your body toward your hands, staying low. Push with your hands as you draw yourself forward and upward into **Cobra**, while widening your collarbones and keeping your elbows tucked right beside your body.

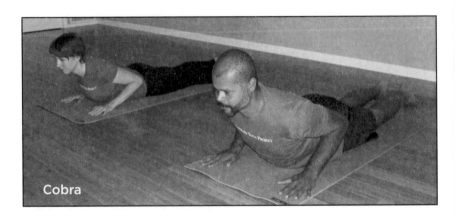
Cobra

Repeat Wisdom Pose and Cobra a few times.

Keeping your hands directly under your shoulders, yield and press your hands fully into the earth, roll your toes under, bend your knees, and press back into **Downward Facing Dog**. From this firm press of your hands see if you can draw your awareness all the way through to your sitting bones and tailbone. Maintain your navel support and a soft bend in your knees. Lengthen both sides of your waist. If you have tight hamstrings, feel free to bend your knees even more.

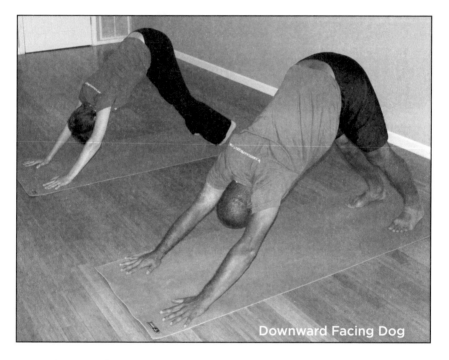

Downward Facing Dog

From here, walk your hands to your feet or your feet to your hands.

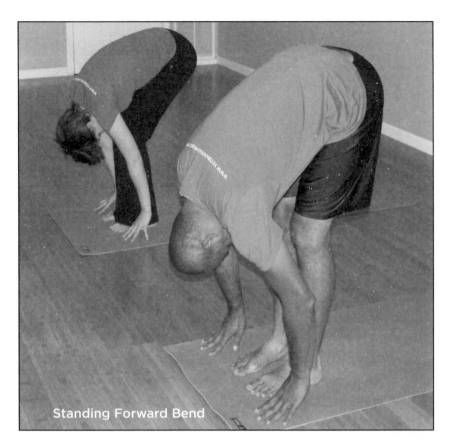

Standing Forward Bend

When you have arrived, exhale all the way over into a **Standing Forward Bend** with your knees bent or soft (not locked).

Inhale and come up to standing, reaching your arms toward the sky, and then exhale your arms down by your sides to **Mountain**. This is a very good place to explore the subtle connections throughout your body.

Spend a couple of minutes here in **Mountain**. Start with your feet hips distance apart. Softening your knees, let the whole bottom of each foot hug the earth. While pressing your feet into the earth, draw your awareness all the way upward through you until you reach the top of your head. Your ankles, hips, and shoulders should all be in a straight line, stacked one over the other. Bring back the imaginary hand on your navel and look for support in that area. An-

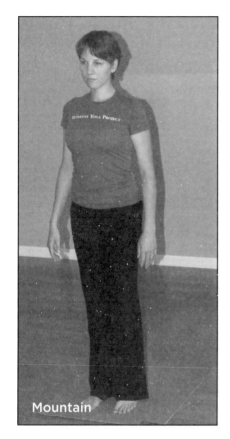

Mountain

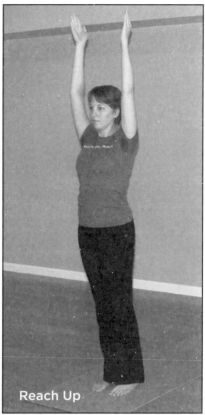

Reach Up

other reminder: try to maintain these supports all the way through the practice. If you forget, it's OK. Practice acceptance and find the supports again.

Stop here and take a few additional breaths. Explore the "Yield" or connection you have with the ground as you press your feet into the earth.

Let's continue to connect movement with breath.

With an inhale, reach through your arms as they rise upward. Exhale and pull them back down by your sides. Fill your body with breath with each inhale. Remember to keep your mouth closed and breathe through your nose as much as possible. *Repeat 3 times.*

Sun Salutation

Begin in **Mountain**.
Press your feet into the earth, inhale and **Reach Up**.

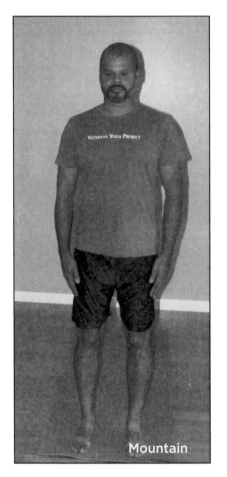

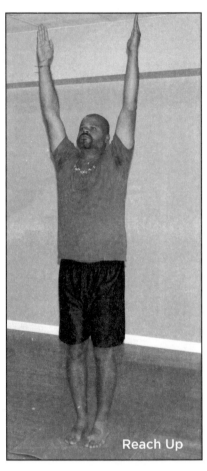

Mountain

Reach Up

Exhale into **Standing Forward Bend,** bending your knees so that you can place your hands on the floor.

On an inhale, maintain navel support as you lengthen out halfway, coming into **Half Standing Forward Bend**.

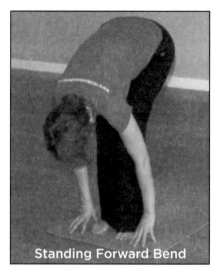

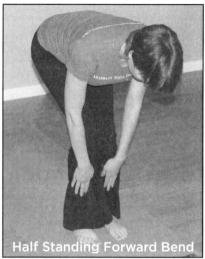

Standing Forward Bend | Half Standing Forward Bend

Bring your hands to the floor, exhale and step back into **Plank**. Your hands should be directly under your shoulders and your body in one long, even line. Feel the press of your hands all the way through to your tailbone and the connection from your feet all the way through to your head. The support in this posture comes from the underside of the body—your navel support. Keep your chest and collarbones wide. Be careful not to let your hips sag toward the earth.

Inhale in **Plank**.

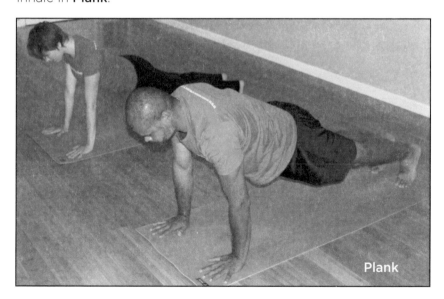

Plank

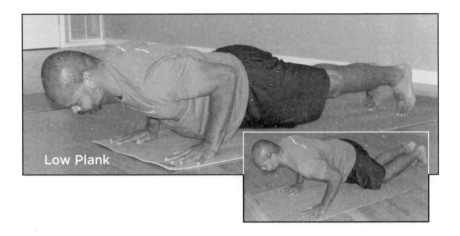

Low Plank

Exhale and lower down halfway to **Low Plank**. Or, you may use the modified version by putting your knees down and lowering your upper body half way down. Be sure to keep your elbows very close to your body and do not let your chest drop lower than your buttocks. This posture can be very challenging.

Inhale your way into **Upward Facing Dog**. The tops of the feet and the hands yield firmly into the earth as you draw yourself forward and upward. This posture is very similar to Cobra except that in Upward Facing Dog the tops of your feet are pressing into the earth and your legs and hips are off the floor. As in Cobra, chest and collarbones remain wide and the support comes from the underside of the body.

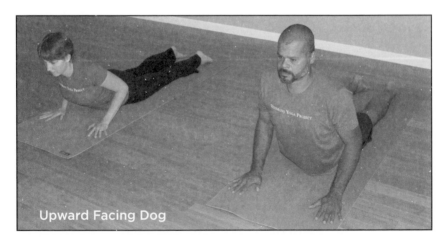

Upward Facing Dog

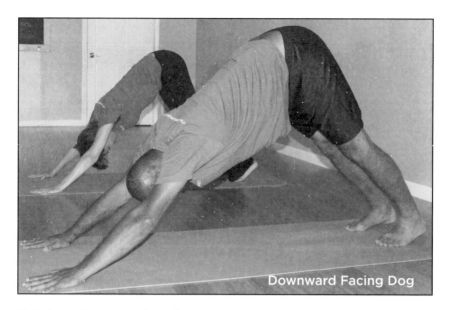
Downward Facing Dog

Exhale to **Downward Facing Dog**. *Take 3-5 breaths here.*

Exhale fully and step your feet forward to your hands. Inhale as you arrive in **Half Standing Forward Bend**. As you reach the crown of your head away, your spine lengthens out into its own neutral curves. Maintaining your navel support will help that. You have the option of keeping your knees soft or even bending them if you feel a tugging on your hamstrings.

Exhale and fold into a **Standing Forward Bend**.

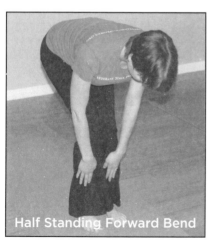
Half Standing Forward Bend

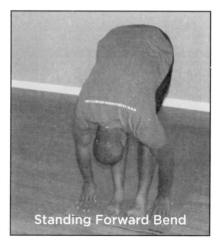
Standing Forward Bend

Inhale and come up **Reaching Up**.

Exhale to **Mountain**.

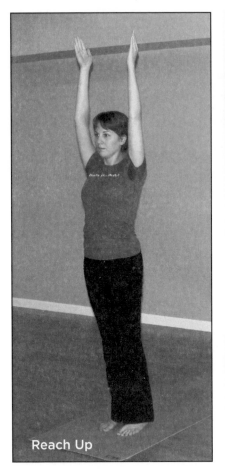

Reach Up

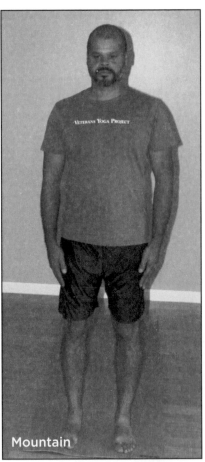

Mountain

Repeat this Sun Salutation 3 times.

Standing Postures

Step out sideways on your mat with your legs a little wider than hips distance. Establish all the same supports that you have used previously to keep you feeling grounded—the press of the feet into the earth and maintaining your navel support.

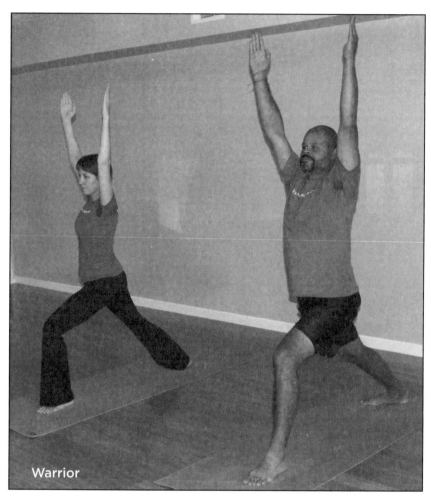

Warrior

Warrior—Begin by spinning your right leg and foot out to the right. Turn your back leg and foot in a little bit. Line up your right heel with the arch of your left foot. Become really planted on the earth through your legs and feet! Inhale and reach your arms over your head. On an exhale, bend your right knee and slide your right sitting bone toward your right foot. Be careful not to let your knee go further forward than your ankle. Stay really stable through your back leg. Remember, this is a very strong and focused posture.

Take 3-5 breaths here. Maintain the supports that keep you grounded. Inhale and push into the earth to straighten your right leg and come out of the posture. Exhale your way back to center. *Repeat this on your left side.*

Triangle—Spin the right leg and foot out again, and be sure to line your feet up in the same way you did in the warrior posture. Inhale and reach your arms out to the sides, and as you exhale lightly bend the right knee. On your next inhale, begin to reach out over your right leg through your right arm—drawing your fingers and hands out and away. As you press your feet into the earth, draw your awareness all the way through to the top of your head. As you exhale, lengthen your right side body out over your right leg.

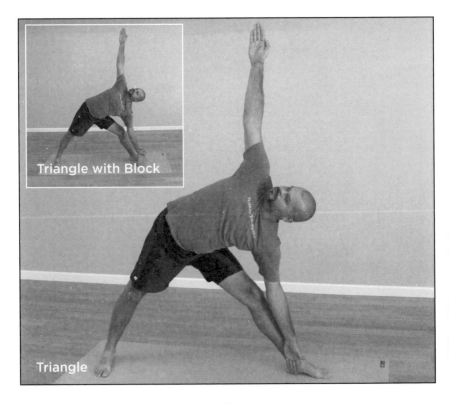

Triangle with Block

Triangle

Extend your right hand down toward your block or your right shin. Let your left arm reach straight up toward the sky, with your left thumb directly over your mouth. *Take 3-5 breaths here.* Then, as you inhale, push into the earth and reach through your arms to come up. Your exhale will bring you back to center. *Repeat on your left side.*

Come back to standing wide-legged on your mat with your feet parallel to the short edge of your mat and a bit wider than your shoulders.

Standing Wide Leg Forward Bend—Place your hands on your hips and take an inhale. Exhale to lengthen your way forward and place your hands on the floor, right between your feet. Inhale and lengthen out half way, and then exhale and fold over. Your hands remain shoulders distance apart. Keep your elbows the same width as your hands. *Take 3-5 breaths here.* Then inhale and lengthen out half way to neutral curves of the spine. Exhale and place your hands on your hips, pressing your feet into the earth and using navel support. Inhale as you come all the way back up.

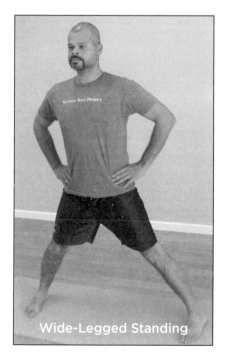

Wide-Legged Standing

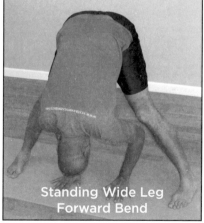

Standing Wide Leg Forward Bend

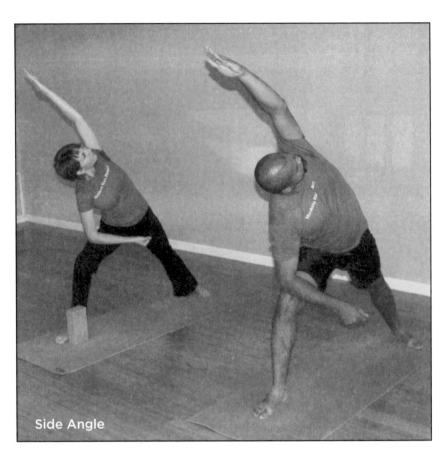

Side Angle

Side Angle and Revolved Side Angle—Repeat the same alignment of your feet as in Warrior and Triangle, beginning on the right side. Inhale and reach your arms out to the sides. As you exhale, bend your right knee. Inhale again. As you exhale, bring your right forearm to your right thigh and reach your left arm all the way over your head for **Side Angle**. Be mindful not to collapse onto your right leg. Maintain the reach of your left arm and the support of the underside of your body. Keep your collarbones wide, so as not to collapse in your chest. *Take 3-5 breaths.* Inhale and come back up to center, going right to next posture on this side.

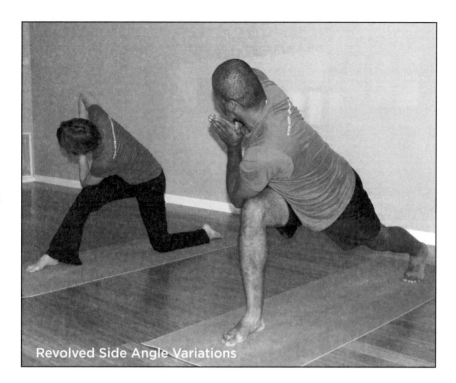

Revolved Side Angle Variations

Exhale, spin your right foot forward, and take your left knee to the earth. As you inhale again, reach your left arm straight up in the air, lengthening the whole left side of your body. Exhale and hook your left elbow around your right knee. Press your palms firmly together and spiral toward the right. You can stay here in a **Revolved Side Angle.** Or you can turn the toes of your left foot under, and bring your left knee up into another variation of **Revolved Side Angle**. *Take 3–5 full breaths here.* Inhale and exhale as you release this posture. Inhale again and come up through center. *Repeat Side Angle and Revolved Side Angle on the other side.*

Balancing

Tree—To balance in a posture it is helpful to be calm, steady, and focused. Remember that your even and steady breath is one of the tools that helps you stay calm and in the present moment.

Keep your gaze fixed on one point to help you be steady and calm. Press both feet firmly into the earth while drawing your awareness up to the crown of your head. Notice whether you still have navel support. Bring your right foot up and press it against your left leg. You can bring your foot above your knee or below your knee. You can even keep your toes on the floor if needed. Be mindful not to press your foot against your knee. Press your foot into your leg and press your leg into your foot. There is that connection or "yield" again. Press your palms together in front of your heart. You can stay here, or you can reach your arms up as if they were limbs on a tree growing toward the sun. Try to stay calm and steady by focusing on your gazing point and your breath, even if your tree sways a little. *Take 5-10 breaths.*

Your exhale brings you back to **Mountain**. *Repeat on the left side.*

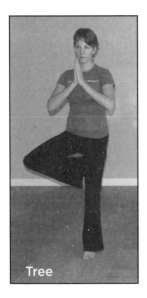
Tree

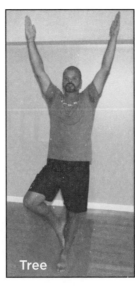
Tree

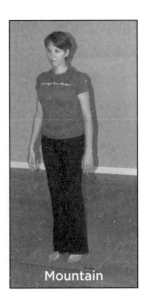
Mountain

From **Mountain**, with your feet pressing into the earth, inhale and reach up. Exhale and fold forward, placing your hands on the floor, and step back into **Plank**. Inhale, and as you exhale this time lower yourself all the way to the floor (belly down).

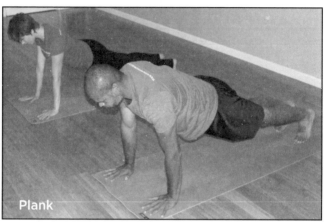

Mountain   Plank

Locust—Extend your arms alongside your body and press the backs of your hands into the earth. Remember to maintain your navel support. This is very important here because it supports the spine from the underside. It should feel as if someone has their hand on your belly and is lightly pressing inward. On the next inhale, lift and extend your feet and upper body at the same time. You are not just lifting your feet and body up—you are extending them in opposite directions. This creates space in the spine. You

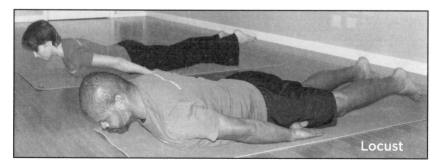

Locust

don't have to lift very high but you should try to reach your head and shoulders in one direction and your feet in the other. Remember to keep your inhale and exhale even. *Take 5 breaths here, then lower down on an exhale. Repeat this 3 times.*

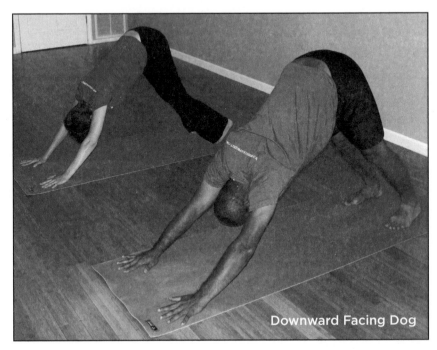

Downward Facing Dog

Press the palms of your hands on the earth under your shoulders, and come to hands and knees. Exhale as you press back into **Downward Facing Dog**. *Take 3–5 breaths.* Inhale and come back to hands and knees, and then come to sitting on your mat.

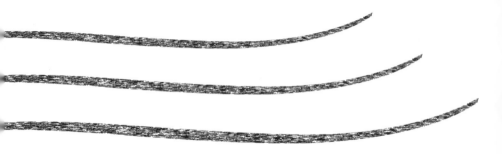

Boat—In a seated position, place both of your feet on the floor. Place your hands behind your knees and lengthen your spine by drawing your awareness up toward the top of your head. Next reach your arms forward, and scoop your belly inward. Lift your feet off the floor and reach them away from you. Do not let your lower back collapse. Keep the crown of your head reaching upward. You may keep your knees bent or extend your legs

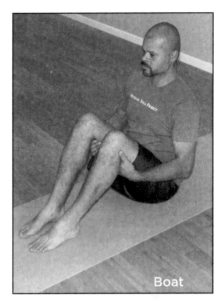

Boat

until your toes are at eye level. If your lower back continues to collapse, just lift one leg. *Take 3-5 breaths.* On an exhale, bring your feet back to the floor. *Repeat. If you are lifting one leg, be sure to lift the other leg the second time.*

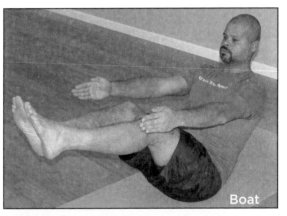

Boat

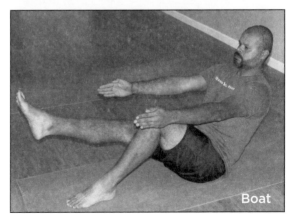

Boat

Seated Half Forward Bend—If you have tight hamstrings you may use a strap in this posture and you may even place a support (such as a blanket) under your sitting bones to lift you slightly. Optimally, you want to be seated right on the center of your sitting bones. Extend your left leg and place your right foot against your left thigh. Press your foot firmly into your thigh and let your thigh press back the same way you did in Tree. Inhale and reach for your left foot or your shin. You can even place a strap around your foot and reach for the strap. This is a really nice variation for tight hamstrings. Maintain the integrity of your spine by reaching through the crown of your head. Try to keep as much length in your spine as possible; it can be really easy to collapse here. Then, as you exhale, fold toward your left leg. *Take 5 breaths here.* Inhale and come back to center and exhale to release. *Repeat on the other side.*

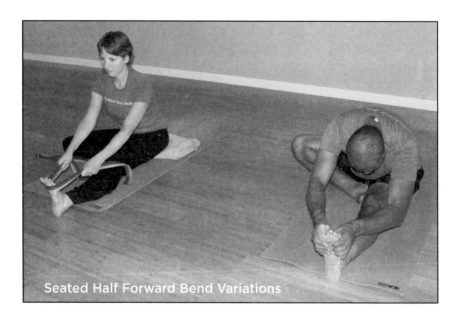

Seated Half Forward Bend Variations

Supported Bridge—Lie down on your back with your feet on the earth and your feet and knees hips distance apart. Draw your heels back toward your sitting bones. Inhale and press your feet into the earth as you press your hips upward. As you bring your hips up and roll onto the tops of your shoulders, place your block under your sacrum. *The sacrum is the solid bone at the base of the spine, below the lumbar curve and between the sacroiliac joints. The block should feel comfortable here.*

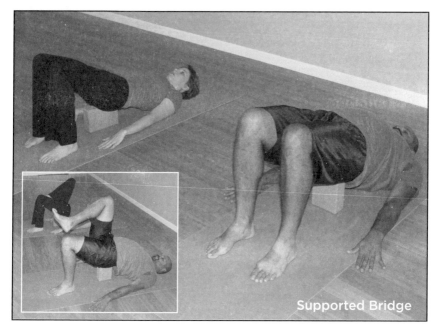

Supported Bridge

The block can be used at three different heights. Flat on its wide side is the lowest height. The skinny long side is the next step up. The skinny short side is the highest.

Once you have the block under your sacrum, place your hands back on the floor alongside your body and press them firmly into the earth. Draw your chin toward your chest and do not turn your head from side to side. Inhale, and as you exhale draw your right knee in toward your chest. On your next inhale extend your right leg straight up in the air. *Take 3-5 breaths here.*

Inhale again, and as you exhale this time draw your right knee back in toward your chest. Your next inhale will bring your right foot back to the earth. Inhale again, and as you exhale draw your left in toward your chest. Inhale and extend your left leg upward. *Take 3–5 breaths here.* Inhale and exhale, drawing your left knee in toward your chest. Leave your left knee here and draw your right knee in as well. Both feet will be off the floor so be sure that you are supporting yourself with your hands as well as the block.

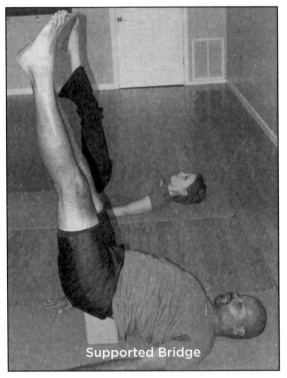

Supported Bridge

The next time you inhale, extend both legs upward. *Take at least 5 breaths here.* After taking the last breath, inhale, then exhale as you draw your knees in toward your chest. Inhale and place both feet back on the floor. Press both feet into the earth and come up just a little higher, then remove the block from under your sacrum. Inhale, reach your arms over your head, and as you exhale lower your back to the floor—one vertebra at a time, starting at the shoulders, and then the mid back, and finally the lower back.

Take a moment here to let your spine settle.

Rest

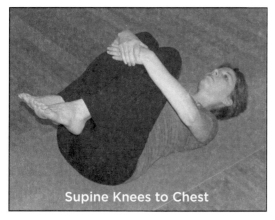
Supine Knees to Chest

Draw your knees in toward your chest again, and wrap your arms around them. With your knees still close to your chest, place your right hand on your left knee and extend your left arm straight out to the left. Inhale, and as you exhale roll your knees to the right. Take several breaths here. Inhale and draw your knees back to center, and exhale as you squeeze them back in toward your chest. Inhale and reach for your right knee with your left hand. Extend your right arm out to the right and exhale your knees all the way over to the left. Take several breaths here. Inhale and bring your knees back to center and squeeze in one more time. Exhale and release your feet to the earth.

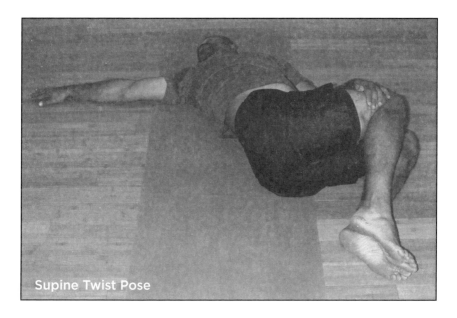
Supine Twist Pose

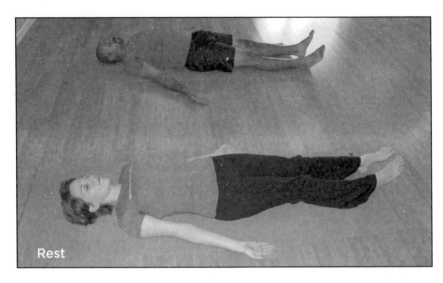

Rest

For rest you may lie on your back with your legs and arms extended, or you may find the posture that is most comfortable for you. If you can close your eyes, you may do so now, or just soften and rest your eyes.

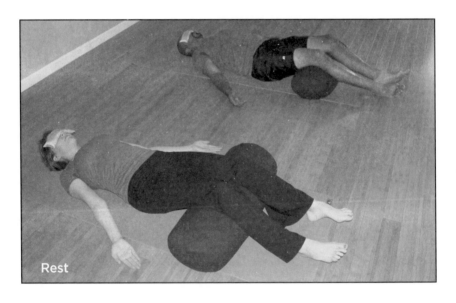

Rest

Spend 5 to 10 minutes resting and absorbing the work you have done.

See practice guide poster inserted into this guide.

Yoga Nidra

Yoga Nidra is a practice that leads us into the deepest level of relaxation in the body and mind. The rest achieved in in the practice of Yoga Nidra can be far more effective than the rest achieved in conventional sleep. The total relaxation achieved in a Yoga Nidra session can be equivalent to hours of ordinary sleep and is profoundly rejuvenating for the body and nervous system. This technique is the jewel of yoga practice and anyone can do it.

The practice is found in the place between sleep and waking. This is a place of clarity where wisdom is uncovered, a place we can learn to be present. Fear arises when we live in the future. The future is only a figment of our imagination. We really don't know what will happen next. Regret and reactiveness arrive from living in the past. The past is now a memory. We can't go back. We can only live in the present. Many of us are stuck in the past or constantly worried about the future. Yoga Nidra helps us access the clarity and wisdom that can help us to stay in the present.

It is common to notice physical shifts or jumps in the body during the practice. This means negative patterns are being released as we tap into our natural, restful wisdom.

Systematic practice of Yoga Nidra may improve the health of the nervous system. The more frequently you use this practice, the more quickly you will notice its effects. A daily practice is highly recommended with the accompanying CD, "**Deep Relaxation: Yoga Nidra with Patty Townsend**". The time of day that you use this practice is completely up to you. Some veterans report better results in the morning and and some veterans report better results in the evening when they cannot sleep.

Yoga Nidra has been used for a multitude of imbalances, ranging from simple relaxation to insomnia, trauma, anxiety, fear, and depression. In order to harmonize our own body and mind, we need to find peace from within. Yoga Nidra is a major key to finding this peace. The modern world is full of overstimulation and we are rewarded for multi-tasking. This ancient practice can be of huge benefit in a modern world.

Please use the accompanying CD, "**Deep Relaxation with Yoga Nidra**" as often as possible. The first track will explain the practice. You may want to listen to it the first time. After you become familiar with it you may skip to the second track, which is the practice itself.

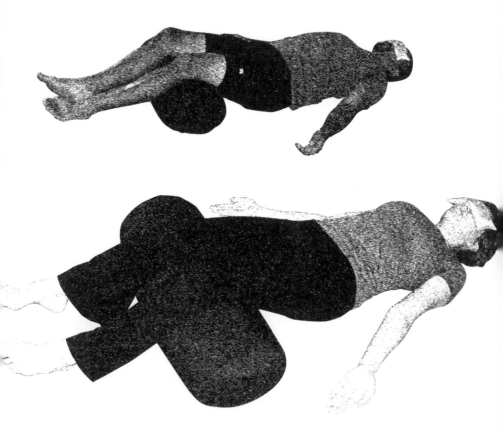

Meditation

Meditation is a practice by which we can become better acquainted with our own mental processes and therefore with our self. The mind can be a great source of distress when it is out of our control. When we cannot slow it down, or direct it, the mind becomes a source of anguish and frustration. The practice of meditation allows us to gain control of this so that we can use it to our benefit instead of allowing it to cause us distress. The practice of meditation allows us to find clarity, peace, and ultimate freedom.

Sample Meditation Practice

Find a comfortable sitting position. You can sit on a cushion on the floor or on a chair. If you sit in a chair, you are encouraged to make sure that your feet are flat on the floor and connecting you to earth. Sit forward on the chair, so that you are not leaning back onto the chair, collapsing your spine, or rounding your low back or shoulders. If you are sitting on the floor, you can sit on a cushion with your legs crossed in front of you, and you can even sit with your back against the wall. What is most important is to find whatever position will allow you to feel comfortable with your spine supported and alert.

Rest your hands wherever it feels best. Options include in your lap, or one hand on each leg.

If you can comfortably close your eyes, please do so. If not, please soften your gaze.

Then, when you are comfortable and ready, bring your complete attention to the sensation of your breath. Feel the breath inside your nostrils. Notice the physical sensations of each inhale and each exhale. You may notice the breath feels cool on the way in and warm on the way out. You may notice it feels soft and fuzzy like cotton or even has a velvety quality.

Just experience this breath and sensation without changing or judging it. Simply observe and accept this experience as it feels right now, in this moment.

At some point it is likely that you will find that your mind has wandered away from the breath. This is to be expected. It is the nature of the mind to wander and its job to think. But we can become aware that the mind has wandered, maybe note where it went, and then gently, non-judgmentally bring our attention back to the inhale and exhale, and the raw sensation of the breath. Instead of judging yourself when you find that the mind has wandered, just simply allow your attention to return back to the breath in this moment.

When you begin this practice, you may start by sitting for 10–15 minutes. Eventually you may want to grow into a 30-minute practice.

There is a sample guided meditation practice on the "**Breathe In, Breathe Out**" CD that accompanies this practice guide.

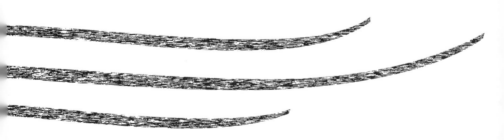

The Practice of Gratitude

This very simple practice starts with just being grateful for what we have in our lives. Try taking a moment each day to acknowledge one thing that you are grateful for. As you practice, your focus will shift. Maybe the glass will be half full instead of half empty.

It may get difficult when life presents its challenges, but this practice can change your outlook and the way that you move through life.

Start by pressing the palms of your hands together in front of your heart. Drop your gaze or take a slight bow with your head. See if this helps you arrive at a place that feels like gratitude. As you arrive there, think of one thing in your life today that you are truly grateful for and acknowledge it silently.

Try to carry this feeling with you throughout your day.

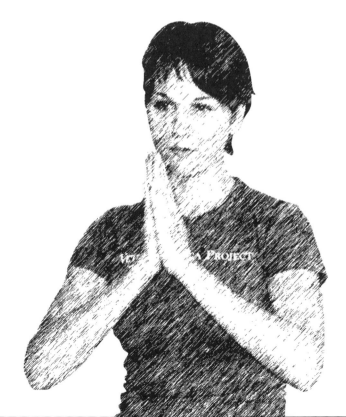

A Final Word

This guide is designed to help you discover the practices of yoga. It's normal to feel skeptical about starting yoga. After all, it's new and unfamiliar. Talking with other veterans who practice yoga, asking questions, and reading or researching online may help you gain a better understanding. You may locate a yoga class for veterans at a local VA or Veterans Center. We also encourage you to try several different yoga classes in your community. There are many different styles of yoga. While one may not resonate with you, another will. Don't be turned off by the ones that don't; keep trying classes and teachers until you find the place that feels correct for you. Once you start a practice, it's important to give it some time; results are not immediate. That's why it's called a practice. The positive results may surprise you and may be well worth the effort.

For resources, visit the Veterans Yoga Project website at www.veteransyogaproject.org.

Glossary

Yoga is taught by many yoga teachers in the language of Sanskrit. We thought it would be helpful to include some of the commonly used words so that if you ever decide to go to a yoga class in your community, you would not feel lost or uncomfortable. Sanskrit is is just another language, nothing creepy.

Yoga is not a religion. However, it does seem to help us find a connection with body, mind, and spirit.

Asana
Asana is the name of the practice of the postures, or the postures connected to breath with movement in a steady and comfortable way.

Namaste
Pronounced *na-ma-stay*. Is usually used as a greeting or when someone is leaving. It means "the light in me honors the light in you."

Om
Om is said to be the sound of the vibration of the universe. Some yoga classes will chant the word Om before or after a class. They are acknowledging the sound of the universe.

Pranayama
The Sanskrit name for the breathing practices. *Prana* means life force or breath of life and *ayama* means to stretch or extend. *Pranayama* is the practice of moving our breath through our body. There are many ways to practice pranayama and in fact Tactical Breathing may be one you are already acquainted with. Some practices are very strong and build heat, and others are softer and calming. The practices in this guide and on your "**Breathe In, Breathe Out**" CD are the pranayama practices we recommend for veterans recovering from PTSD.

Ujjayi

A type of pranayama or breathing practice. *Ujjayi* means "victorious" but sometimes is called "Ocean Breath" because it sounds like the ocean. This sound is made by creating a slight constriction at the back of the throat while the mouth is closed. By doing this we are able to sip the breath in slowly and create better absorption and balance in the nervous system. You are encouraged to create an even length for the inhale and the exhale. You want to breathe in as much breath as you breathe out.

Yoga

The word *yoga* means "union." It's an ancient discipline that consists of many practices including breathing practices, movement and postures, yoga nidra, meditation and mindfulness. It is not a religion or an exercise program. As we learn to direct the breath, body, and mind, we begin to unite them, become whole, and find peace.

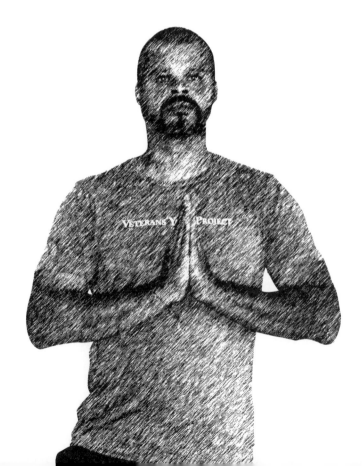

Mindful Movement Asana Practice (Pictures Only)

Below is the mindful movement asana practice presented in pictures only. As you become familiar with the practice, you may want to use just these pictures to guide you.

Moving Warm-Up

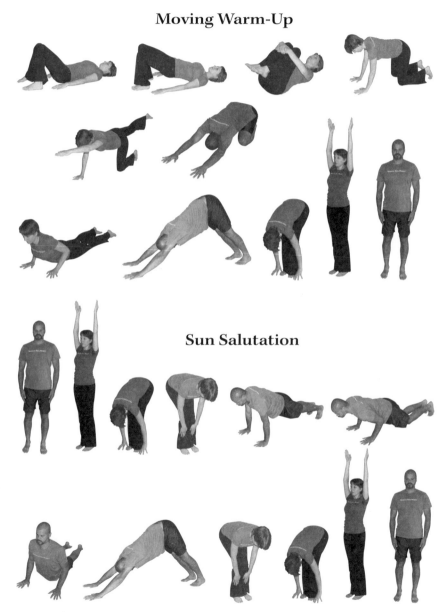

Sun Salutation

Practice the rows of postures from left to right.

Standing Postures

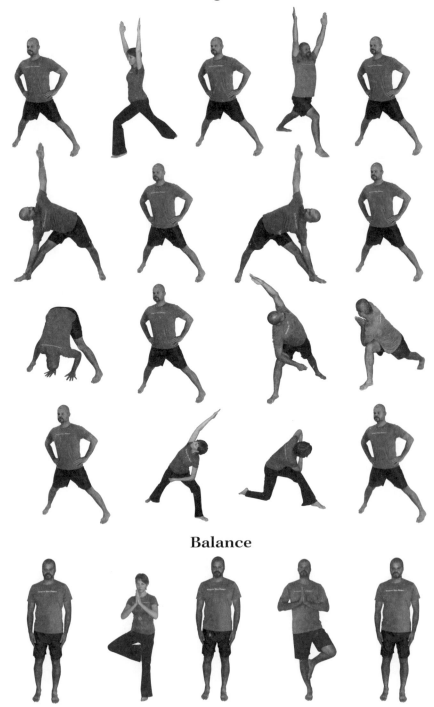

Balance

Seated and Reclined Postures

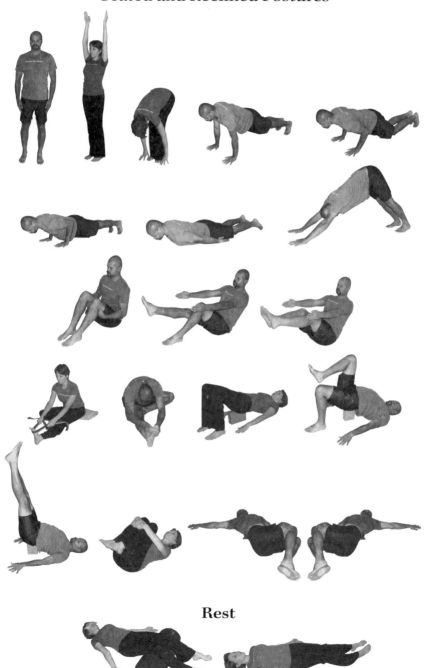

Rest

Practice the rows of postures from left to right.

65

About the Authors and Co-Founders
of the Veterans Yoga Project

Suzanne Manafort, ERYT-50. Director of Newington Yoga Center is a member of the International Association of Yoga Therapists. She studied at Yoga Center Amherst with Patty Townsend, completing her 500-hour program in Embodyoga®. She also completed a 500-hour program with Beryl Bender Birch and a teacher training with David Swenson. Most recently, Suzanne has deepened her meditation practice, studying with Pandit Rajmani Tigunait at the Himalayan Institute in The Living Tantra Program.

Suzanne has been teaching yoga to Veterans coping with combat-related PTS in a PTS Residential Rehabilitation Program for several years and also teaches groups for women veterans in an outpatient PTS program. In 2009, she was designated a Wells Fargo Second Half ChampionÐ for her work with Veterans. Suzanne also serves on the board of directors of the Give Back Yoga Foundation.

Daniel J. Libby is a licensed clinical psychologist specializing in the integration of evidence-based psychotherapies and Complementary and Alternative Medicine practices for the treatment of PTS and other psychological and emotional distress in active-duty military and veterans.

As a Postdoctoral Fellow with Yale University's Department of Psychiatry and the VA's Mental Illness Research and Education Clinical Center, Daniel conducted research investigating the neural correlates of mindfulness meditation as well as the first epidemiological investigation of Complementary and Alternative Medicine in VA PTSD treatment programs.

Daniel is now in private practice providing clinical and consulting psychological services for veterans and the organizations that serve them. He is also a graduate of the 200-hour embodyoga® Teacher Training and serves as President of the Board of Directors of the Feathered Pipe Foundation, the extraordinary nonprofit educational foundation and yoga retreat center.

Testimonials

I was introduced to yoga during my time at the PTSD Rehabilitation Residential Program in Newington, CT. The Veterans Yoga Program has been incredibly helpful to me in coping with my PTSD. Yoga is like a gyro that brings me back into equilibrium when dealing with the effects of my disorder. The more I practice, the more my symptoms are mitigated. Yoga has helped to reduce my anxiety and has improved my ability to focus. I like the challenge of doing something that tests my abilities and rewards me with observable progress which keeps me motivated. I think of Yoga as survival training for the veteran's mind, body, and soul.

—Paul, Vietnam War Veteran

I teach yoga for veterans at the VA in Topeka, Kansas. The VA has a 24 bed/7 week program. The Mindful Yoga Therapy for Veterans Coping with Trauma book and the 2 CD's have been helpful with information about Post Traumatic Stress (PTS). It describes PTS and gives you a toolbox to help veterans break the cycle with breathing techniques, mindful movement with a practice guide, Yoga Nidra, Meditation and Gratitude. It is concisely written with great information. The CDs that come with it are well done and helpful for my classes.   *—Sidney*

I wanted to take a moment to thank you and the organization for the CDs and Veterans Yoga Project practice guide. The audio CDs were great quality, and I think they would be an asset to any Vet or active duty service member looking to use pranayama and yoga nidra as tools in managing PTSD or other trauma. We've been working with Vets in Houston for over two years, and looking to increase our footprint very soon. Harris county (Houston's location) has the second highest population of military Veterans in the US, and our VA medical center is one of the largest anywhere. So, we have a significant population here that needs our help. Thanks again for your interest and great work in this community.

—Carl Salazar, Founder and Executive Director of Expedition Balance.

"Yoga has helped my racing mind stop racing".

—Heather, Iraqi War Veteran

"Yoga Nidra helps me access the true me."   *—Diane, Saigon 70*

"Yoga and this practice guide is my personal pathway to paradise."
—D,Veteran

"Mindful Yoga Therapy brings clarity to my life." —Veteran

My name is Sandra. I've been part of the Canadian Forces family for the past 26 years, including my husband Eric, children Sarah and Patrick. As any family in the military, we've gone through a lot of changes, emotional ups and downs, and worries. The first time I heard my husband was going on a mission for 6 months, I began feeling a lot of stress. We'd never gone through a separation for that long. I started reading books on how to cut stress out of my life.

The information that I was looking for at the time is being given to you in the palm of your hands. The only thing you need to do is the practice. These techniques in Mindful Yoga Therapy are simple and powerful. For example: "Deep breathing sends a message to the brain that all is well and cuts the stress cycle." Wow, with the breathing practice I realized that I didn't need to be in a relaxed atmosphere to reduce stress. It's that simple. I started to take time every day even if I only had a minute to spare and say to myself "am I breathing in, and breathing out?" Some days that is all I needed to feel calm again.

If you would like to introduce some thing in your life that is simple but powerful that will change your life, this toolkit from the Veteran's Yoga Project is a very good starter kit. It has worked for me and still is keeping me balanced and calm. If you open up to this program you will see positive results in no time! —Sandra Woods-Poulin

I highly recommend The Practice Manual to any veteran past, present, or future. PTSD is becoming prevalent among the men and women who graciously serve our country. This practice manual can be a great instrument in understanding PTSD and how yoga and mindfulness can integrate into healing modalities. There are detailed descriptions of each practice with alternatives in this easy to use manual developed for all veterans.
—Ann Richardson, CYI, E-RYT, Owner and Director of Studio Bamboo Institute of Yoga serving wounded, ill, and injured through Adaptive Yoga